TAYLOR DINES

Escaping The Light

Escape the light and find peace in the darkness

First edition

Editing by Bradley Charbonneau

This book was professionally typeset on Reedsy.
Find out more at reedsy.com

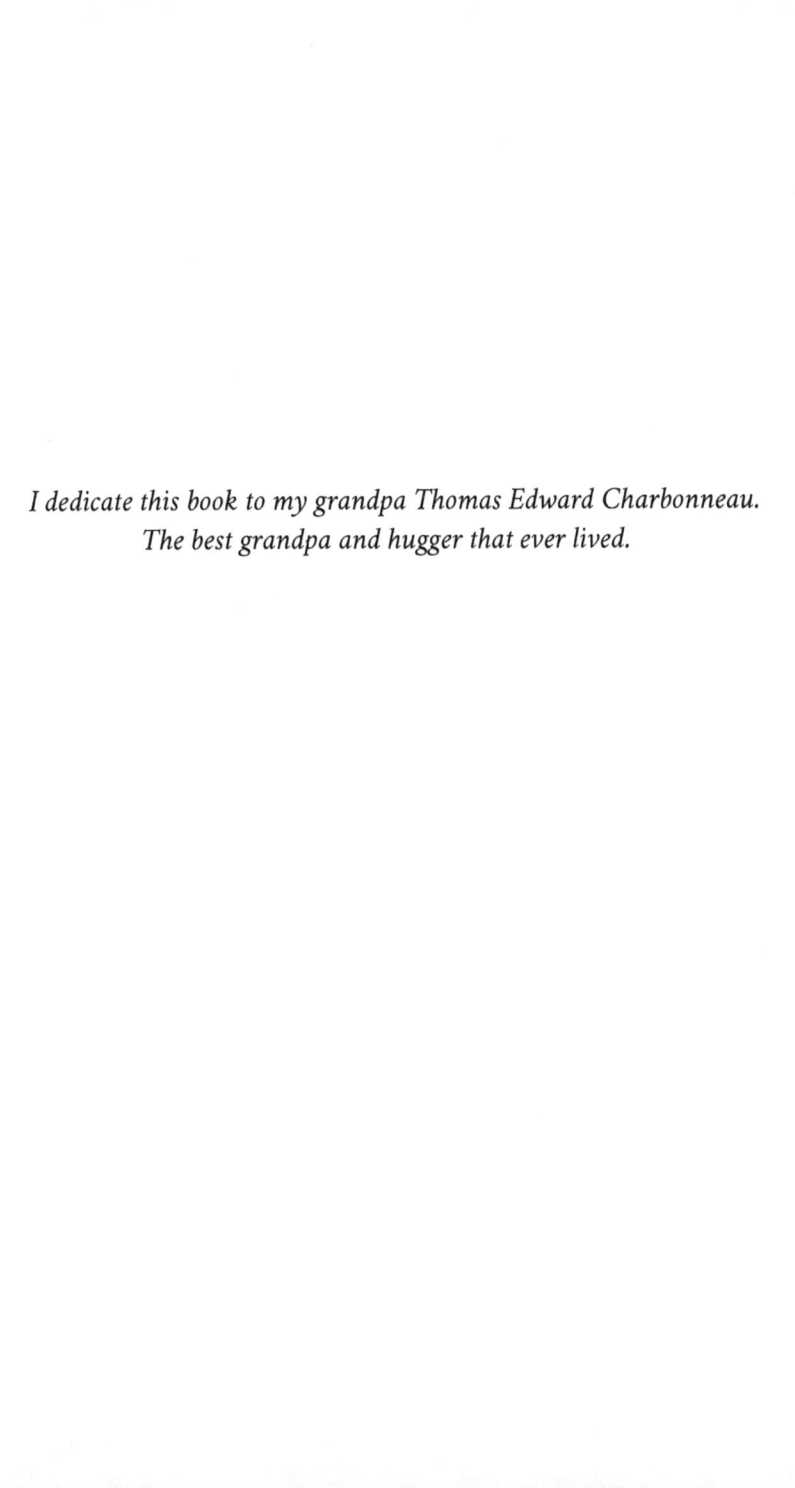

I dedicate this book to my grandpa Thomas Edward Charbonneau.
The best grandpa and hugger that ever lived.

Contents

V What

Foreword

"No matter how busy you are, you should make the time, even if it is just 10 minutes, to sit or lie with your eyes closed in peace." — *Taylor Dines*

The book you have in your hands in Taylor Dines' worst book.

It's her best book.

Both are true because it's also her first book.

Did you ever go to the bank or listen to your grandfather tell you that if you had just put away that money 47 years previous that today you would have compound interest and enough to buy a cruise to Alaska?

He shakes his head and sighs in the lost opportunity. Why didn't he tell you that 47 years ago?

Let's say today is 47 years in the past from 47 years in the future. Are you still with me? It's the present day. What we do today will alter the trajectory of our future. What we do today will affect us 47 years from now.

Taylor Dines is writing about how a 10-minute nap (with the aid of an eye mask) can boost your productivity, rejuvenate your energy, and is better than a 3-hour snooze. If you take her advice and start today, you could improve your health, deepen your sleep, and, who knows, live longer—maybe go on that cruise in 47 years.

What Taylor is also doing today is writing her first book.

I hope it's her worst book. Why? Because with each book she improves. Each time she writes, she learns something. Every subsequent book takes the experience, the feedback, and the learning of each previous book and she gets smarter, faster, better.

But she has to begin.

This is her beginning.

I run a workshop called Spark Campfire where an adult (in this case, me) co-creates a book together with a younger person. The adult might be an uncle, a grandmother, or...you.

The younger person might be a 9-year-old girl, a monosyllabic-15-year-old teen (I have a ripe specimen in my laboratory...), or...your nephew.

It's not unlike grandpa advising you to invest your money so it earns compound interest over the long run. If we start now, if we, for example, use our creativity to write a book when we're young, we don't lose that experience. In fact, just like the money, it builds exponentially not just because we started early, but because we started at all.

Do you know what $0 looks like after 47 years? Yep, still $0.

Do you know what a 17-year-old girl gets from writing (and publishing) a book after 47 years?

Either do I, but it's going to be greater than zero, more than nothing, and if I were a betting man, I'd bet her experience here grows exponentially, unexpectedly, and in ways she will only know because she did it, she started, she took that first step.

You have that first step in your hands.

If you happen to run across Taylor, please shake her hand. Congratulate her on completing her first book, pat her on the back for taking that first step, and let her know if she might have had the slightest influence on you and your sleep habits and maybe she helped you get even just one better night's sleep.

But by buying this book, by sharing it with friends, by helping support a young person who's taking her first steps into the world, you're backing her creativity, you're encouraging her to dare to get out of her comfort zone and put her words into this book and out to the public.

You're confirming what I have learned over the course of our working together. Taylor Dines has the guts to share her thoughts with strangers. She has the stamina to write the words that fill the empty pages. She didn't just take the many steps it took to finish, she took the hardest step of all: the first step.

If you see her in passing some day, please whisper into her ear: *Taylor Dines is a rockstar.*

Bradley Charbonneau
Author and Founder of Spark Campfire
Driebergen, The Netherlands
June 2019

Preface

"Happiness can only be found if you can free yourself of all other distractions." -Saul Bellow

Think about this: you sleep on average about eight hours a day, that is 1/3 of a full day. In one year, you will sleep 2,920 hours, which is about 121 days of sleep. Imagine how much you sleep in a lifetime.

Sleep matters, so how can you make it better?

I

Who

1

My way

Y ou are here, reading this book, for a reason. You are reading this because you are attempting to find a solution to your problem, sleep. You can do it my way or your way. You may even pick little snippets out of my way and create your own way.

So what is my way?

My way involves an eye mask. Most people wouldn't think of this solution right off the bat. People usually go for dark curtains or attempting to cover every light source in your bedroom. My way allows you to sleep in the brightest places.

This amazing invention is similar to putting a pillow over your head in the morning when the light is bright and you want it to go away. This way is a pillow for your eyes. This little contraption will change your sleeping life forever.

You can bring it anywhere, and sleep like it's the middle of the night, but when it's actually the middle of the day. The best thing about this sleeping mask is that you don't have to use it all the time. Some people only use it for when they travel. I wear it every night to sleep. It's all up to you, you can wear it all the time or just on certain occasions. You can also choose to wear it just in the morning when the light streaming through your windows wakes you up. My way—any time you need to sleep, slip it on, and boom, you're out.

2

Not my way, your way

*"My parents used to play me this album when I couldn't
go to sleep. It was called 'Deep Forest.' I think it was
a self-titled record. It's actually still one of my favorite
albums of all time."*
-Flume

Your way:
Everyone has different situations. Analyze the origin
of this problem, whether it be noisy or jumping from
one house to another, a lumpy bed on a camping trip, a sleeping
mask will block out all of the things that make you feel like
you are somewhere else. Your way is different, you can add
or change anything. For instance, some people like going to
bed with some sort of white noise or music making them fall
deeper into sleep.

However, most teens are thinking about everything that
happened to them during the day, or even worrying or being

nervous about something that is coming in the next day, this will hinder your ability to fall asleep quickly. **Since there is no way to really wipe your mind of thoughts, the best thing you can do is try to push away the nagging thoughts that keep creeping into your mind.** Everyone really has their own way of attempting to do this. For example, when you were little, you were often told to count the cows jumping over the moon, or to count your breathes until you doze off into a deep slumber. Focusing on one thing will do you better than focusing on the million other things in the world.

II

Why?

3

Teenage Addiction

Teenagers aren't taught to meditate or take a moment to focus on themselves for even 15 seconds.

While adults have more experience with stress, distractions, they have more resources than teenagers do. A sleeping mask can be a way for teenagers to cope with distractions and runaway thoughts. A first step towards a way to eliminate distractions of the world for a little while.

However, there is a serious epidemic common among teens: social media and phone usage. I could go into all the different problems with this like the blue light in the phone, the fact that one comment on a picture can live in your mind for days, and so much more, but I won't.

"I can't go to sleep without being near a plug," a very good friend told me last week.

This is a good example of never being fully asleep, she will always be semi-awake, waiting for that phone to buzz.

Addiction is defined as:

Persistent compulsive use of a device known by the user

to be potentially harmful. (Merriam-Webster)

She is addicted to her phone. So why is this a bad thing? How will this affect her life? She is relying on other people's opinions instead of being confident in herself. She is living in a virtual world, not reality.

"Technology is neutral, it depends on how it's used."
  - Rick Smolan

4

Should I try this?

There's so many things running through your mind. If you can formulate a game plan that works for you and allows you to block outside distractions and get to what matters, that's how the talent is able to come out.
-Jake Arrieta

An eye mask is a game changer. If you are someone who likes to take naps, this will be your best friend. I encourage you to try it even if you think it is stupid. It was the best $7 I ever spent! You can try and spend money on other little things that you think might help, but this is the one thing you are missing. And if you truly do not like it, you can keep it for travels, when you can't cover up the light in places like an airplane.

5

10 minutes

One way to boost our will power and focus is to manage
our distractions instead of letting them manage us.
-Daniel Goleman

Whats 10 minutes out of 24 hours?
It's worth trying…. A 10 minute break can be more influential than a 3-hour break. Studies show that 10 minutes will do more for your body than 30 minutes or 3 hours. After 30 minutes your body will fall into a deeper sleep called sleep inertia. Sleep inertia is when you wake up feeling drowsy and groggy. A 10 minute nap shows immediate solutions beginning with rejuvenation.

Another factor applied this 10 minute nap is the timing of the day. If you nap later in the day, it will mess up your sleep pattern and you will most likely not have a good night sleep. Studies recommend that you nap in the late morning, or the middle of the day. This will give you a boost to get you through the rest of the day!

Another plus is having your eye mask on.

If you are struggling to fall asleep or take a nap, some people are tempted to just get on their phone... an eye mask will keep you from looking at these things and have a deeper focus on falling into a deeper sleep.

III

When & Where

6

My Story

"If you see someone on a plane with an eye mask, sleeping, that's probably me, because that's pretty much where I live." -Ronna McDaniel

My story began with my first flight to Europe. Walking onto the plane I expected horrible food and uncomfortable seats that I wouldn't be able to sleep in, but I expected good movies. When I got to my seat, I had a pillow, blanket, earplugs, and an eye mask waiting for me. I thought to myself "Wow! I didn't expect that!" On my flight, I realized the food was actually good, the movies are juicy, and the eye masks are a lifesaver. One thing I didn't realize is that my sleeping habits would change forever after this day.

Everywhere I went I brought that plane eye mask with me. It made it easier to be able to take naps, and sleep when others wanted to stay up and read with a shining light. I wore it to sleep every night after that plane ride, as it blocked out the thousands of lights streaming through the curtains. On one of my stops in Europe, my beloved eye mask broke… Thank goodness my family kept theirs from the flight, so I had a backup at the ready. That backup eye mask lasted me through the rest of our trip.

On the plane ride back to my home, I received another eye mask, which put a big smile on my face. When I got home, I started to do my research on eye masks. I looked at different material, shapes, sizes, everything you could think of. There are an absurd amount of different types of eye masks, if you take the time to look… Personally, I like a little space above my eyes so I don't feel that they are being pried shut. So, I bought the eye mask that in some ways looks like bug eyes. It allowed me to open my eyes if I *really* needed to, while allowing me to escape into the darkness. The beauty of an eye mask is that it allows me to sleep in while allowing me to feel like it's the middle of the night, pitch black.

At home, I have four large windows in my room that flood with light in the earliest hours of the day, which isn't nice if you are wanting to sleep in. An eye mask was the perfect solution, I just didn't realize it until that one plane ride.

7

When is it "right"?

"One way to boost our will power and focus is to manage our distractions instead of letting them manage us."
-Daniel Goleman

The first time I needed an eye mask, and didn't realize it, was when I was a little girl trying to block out the sun on long road trips. I would hang sweatshirts on the window desperately trying to shut out the light long enough to take a quick nap.... Now, I slip my sleeping mask in my bag so I am ready to sleep in the car like it is the middle of the night.

When would a sleeping mask be right for you?
- Is your room dark enough?
- Is there light coming from the alarm clock?
- Is the light too bright to stay asleep in the morning?

There is no "right" time...

But there is a wrong time (in math class) - your teacher won't understand the value of this brain booster. Studies show that naps improve your productivity. No wonder I see so many people sleeping in class!

Another wrong time is when you are not in a 100% safe place, this could be in a park or bus station, somewhere you are not comfortable. Save your eye mask for a safe and cozy spot to sneak into the land of dreams.

Find those stolen moments, such as a quick trip to your car, where you slip on that eye mask and just sit in peace for a couple minutes. The best time to do this, would possibly be before a test or after an argument with a friend. This is a way for you to relax your body and mind.

Sleeping in a car as a little girl was frustrating. Now, I slip my handy dandy sleeping mask on and I'm ready to sleep!

8

Day Time

In my next life, I want to be a housecat. Naps all the time!
-Laura Anne Gilman

NAPS!
The greatest thing in the world. Just a simple break will do so much for you. A nap doesn't mean sleeping for 2 or 3 hours at a time. A nap is a small break for your body and mind, allowing you to fully relax and get just the right amount of sleep to be rejuvenated.

Many things go on during the day, you work, eat, drive, walk, talk with friends and family, and so much more. Just think of your routine during the day, how much you actually do. If you choose to, you can make time to recharge your batteries.

IV

How

9

Relaxation time matters

I spent a lot of my teenage years experimenting with who
I was as a person and not really getting it right. And then,
I think, I realized that I just had to chill out in life.
  -Charli XCX

You should set goals for yourself every day. It keeps you motivated and less stressed. In this list you should make sure you have down time. No matter how busy you are, you should make the time, even if it is just 10 minutes, to sit or lie with your eyes closed in peace.

This is especially important if you are busy all day long, your body needs to rejuvenate. This is just one more reason I bring my eye mask literally every where I go. It is so easy to slip it on going from one place to the next (if I am not driving of course). One thing teenagers especially need to learn how to do is take care of yourself, putting yourself first.

If you know you have been overworking yourself, reward yourself with some deserved time with your bed. It is not a bad thing to rest or take naps, your body will thank you.

V

What

10

Choices

Everyone is different, so I suggest starting by looking on the internet or going into a normal shop and feeling the texture of each mask and also trying on all the different shapes and sizes. Think about things such as:

1. What type of material?
2. Do you want some space between your eyes and your eye mask?
3. What type of mask would irritate you?

When trying to find my perfect fit, I went through at least 3 different eye masks. I realized that I liked some room between my eyes and the eye mask. Being able to have the darkness without having something pressing and bothering my eyes. Another thing to consider is if you want your nose to be covered or not. This is 100% a personal preference. I personally do not like it because I feel that it bothers my nose.

The two links below, are what I was talking about when I said space above the eyes, not pressing right on your eyes.

https://amzn.to/2F5bT3e

This is a link to a very common eye mask. This eye mask provides space for your eyes and does not pressure them, unless your adjustable strap is very tight. This particular eye mask DOES cover your nose, some may like this. Also, some say that is keeps the light from peeking inside if the eye mask does move at all.

https://amzn.to/2KMVkMV

This is a link to the eye mask that I use. It has space between the eye mask and your eyes, enough that you could open your eyes if you really wanted to. This particular eye mask doesn't cover your nose, which I personally prefer. It also comes with an adjustable strap, a case, and some handy dandy ear buds if you want to escape the noise too!

This is a visual block, sometimes you need an audio block, put some ear buds in and listen to soothing music that doesn't have any lyrics. Any type of way to escape the world and fall into sleep is worth the effort. The bottom line, is to escape the light and find peace in the darkness.

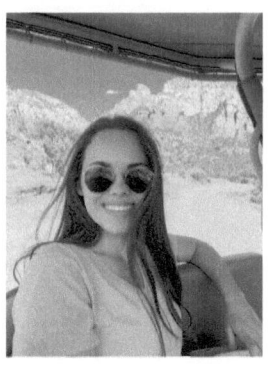

About the Author

My name is Taylor Dines. I am a 17 year old girl who just graduated high school, and am writing my first book! This book was a gift from my uncle, Bradley Charbonneau. For Christmas, his gift to me was to write a book together. This gift made us talk, connect, and grow closer. He will forever be my inspiration for this book.